WORKOUTS

At-Home At-Work 365:

The Most Effective, Convenient, and FREE Workouts on the Planet and Get Ultimate Results

Christopher J. Davis, M.D.

Anna G Taylor

Table of Contents

INTRODUCTION

Congratulations on downloading *Workouts At-Home At-Work 365: The Most Effective, Convenient and FREE Workouts on the Planet and Get Ultimate Results* and thank you for doing so. By purchasing this book, you are already one step closer to reaching your fitness goals in a way that's guaranteed to work and is free! It doesn't get much better than that.

This book will teach you not only great workouts that you can do at home and even while you're at work, but it will also provide you with information on how you can lead a life of strength and happiness through the development of a healthy mindset. Even if you spend your time working out like fiend and see physical results on your body, if you don't have a mindset that is consistent and driven then it's going to be much harder to maintain results in the long-term. This book will help you to develop the mindset that you need to not only see results, but keep these results as well.

The following chapters will discuss many different types of workouts that can complement a busy and chaotic lifestyle. What's especially unique about the workouts that will be presented in this book is that you don't need any special equipment in order to do them. Sure, having a yoga mat might be beneficial to you when we talk about the benefits of yoga; however, even owning a yoga mat at first is not completely necessary.

The point of these workouts is that you should be able to do them essentially anywhere that you feel most comfortable. The takeaway feeling from this book should be an awareness of the fact that you don't need an expensive gym trainer or a hefty monthly gym payment in order to see and feel concrete results. All that you need is already within you; you simply need to cultivate your potential in a way that is efficient, strong, and disciplined.

Thanks again for choosing this one! Every effort was made to ensure it is full of as much useful information as possible, please enjoy!

Chapter 1: A Foolproof Deskercise Routine

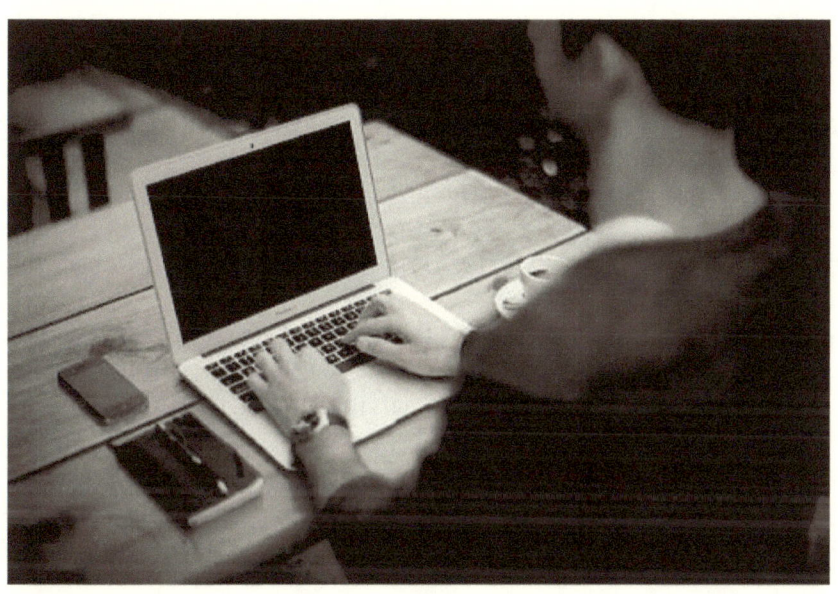

This chapter is going to provide you with a comprehensive workout routine that you can use while you're at work and at your desk. The truth of the matter is that when you sit at your desk all day long, you are hurting your body in numerous ways. Firstly, you are hurting your posture because you are constantly leaning into your computer in hopes of seeing your computer screen as clearly as possible.

Secondly, if you type a lot you are hurting your wrists because of all the typing that you do day in and day out. Three, you are hurting your legs because when you are stationary and in a seated position for a long period of time the muscles in your legs begin to deteriorate rapidly. It's time to get moving in the office! Yes, after learning this deskercise routine you are definitely going to be that crazy man or woman in the office, but who cares!

If you engage in the deskercise routine that is presented in this chapter, you'll have something that your co-workers will not have, and that's strength and your overall long-term health.

Deskercise Tactic 1: Toe Taps

A basic yet effective exercise that is inconspicuous are toe taps that you can do underneath of your desk. For this basic version of the exercise, all that you have to do is rapidly tap one foot and then the other for up to two minutes at a time before taking a rest for one minute.

If you want to get a bit fancier and you don't care about whether or not other people are going to smirk and point at you, a more advanced version of this exercise is to stand behind a small trash can. After you're standing behind the trashcan, pick up your foot so that it taps the edge of the can. Then, bring this foot down and tap the edge of the can with your other foot. Alternate between both feet about ten times.

Deskercise Tactic 2: The Modified Stair Master

If you have an elevator at your office, a great idea to get some exercise at the beginning or end of the day or during your lunch break is to take the stars instead of the elevator. This can seem daunting, especially if you work on a floor that's more than ten floors away; however, stairs are one of the toughest workouts that you can put your body through. Stairs help your cardio, your breathing, and your leg muscles all at the same time. From an exercise standpoint, it doesn't get much more comprehensive than that.

Deskercise Tactic 3: Jogging in Place

Again, this deskercise tactic is for the brave soul who does not care about what their coworkers think of them. Not only does it get boring sitting at a desk all day long, but it can get oddly tiring too. Instead of keeping your eyelids open with paperclips, why not get up for a moment or two and jog in place?

If you want to make it even more tricky for yourself, start by jogging in place and then moving to jogging in place with high knees. This can be done for a minute or two before you hunker down and get back to what you were originally working on. You can also perform this exercise multiple times throughout the day.

Deskercise Tactic 4: Wander

Who says that you don't have to wander towards the bathroom at least twelve times a day or more? Hey, if you drink a lot of water and stay properly hydrated, this will probably be true anyway.

If you work in an environment where you know you won't get in trouble for wandering around, then why not take some liberty doing so? Walk around the office, see what's going on in the kitchen and with your friend who works in another part of the establishment. Of course, when you wander you want to make sure that you're not wandering towards the donuts that are in the conference room, but wandering can be a great way to burn a few calories that would otherwise be turning into fat at your desk.

Deskercise Tactic 5: Desk Squat!

After you've wandered around the office and have successfully distracted your fellow employees, consider removing the chair from your desk and squatting at your computer instead.

This type of squat is the same type of squat that we discussed earlier in the book; however, this time both of the legs are together. When you bend your knees to "sit" down, you should look like you're sitting in a chair.

The legs should be at a ninety-degree angle, and resist the urge to hold onto the desk in front of you. If you do hold onto the desk or onto the arms of the chair behind you, this is basically defeating the purpose of the exercise altogether.

Deskercise Tactic 6: Dips

No, this deskercise tactic does not involve eating tasty dips at your desk, but I know that you probably wish that it did. If you work in a cubicle, there's no reason why you can't work out your arms throughout the day without spending any money or getting on the ground to do some pushups.

Begin by facing away from the desk and grip the desk so that your fingers are underneath of it.

Next, with your legs either out straight or bent slightly, begin to bend your elbows so that they form a ninety-degree angle with the desk. When you've dipped to this point, then begin to straighten your arms once more. Continue this activity for between twenty-five to thirty reps. If you're feeling up to it, try to do this exercise twice a day. You can do exercises such as core workouts at home, but sometimes arms are an area of the body that are overlooked.

Your cubicle dip can be one workout that will force you to tone your arms throughout the day, while you're getting paid!

Deskercise Tactic 7: The Stapler Curl

The last deskercise tactic at which we're going to look is known as the stapler curl. For this tactic, start by placing the stapler in either your left or right hand and with your arm straight begin to bend the forearm until the stapler is touching the upper part of your arm.

After this, begin to lower the forearm once more until your arm is straight again. Continue this for about thirty reps on each side of the body. If a stapler is not heavy enough for you, consider instead lifting a heavy water bottle or even a heavy canister of some kind. Don't be afraid to get creative.

For all of the tactics that were presented in this chapter, it's important to understand that you may be surprised with the results that you see in your body, especially if you are replacing other fattening activity with exercising while at the office. For example, maybe instead of taking that soda break you replace it with doing your arm curls or your desk squats. Maybe instead of pulling out your cookies at 2 P.M., you wander around the office and find people to interact with instead.

Changing your office habits will force you to look at where your habits could improve inside of the office. Of course, some people may look at you funny, but won't that just make this type of lifestyle change even more fun? There's more of a chance that the relaxed and less uptight coworkers that you have may even eventually join in on the fun that you're having.

 If you can get more people to participate in strengthening their body, individual success is much greater.

Chapter 2: How to Exercise at Home in Ten Minutes or Less

If instead of working out at the office, you're someone who enjoys a bit more privacy, then a great alternative is to work out in your home.

If you're a stay a home parent or work from home, you may find that it can be hard to find the time to get a full workout in throughout the day; however, if you think about working out in a different manner, this may become easier for you.

Instead of thinking that you need to workout for thirty or sixty minutes, you can find ten minutes here and there throughout the day to really make your workouts coincide with your busy home schedule. This chapter will look at the types of exercises that you can do at home on a small budget and with little time to spare!

At-Home Workout 1: Stair Step Ups with Knee Raises

Having stairs in your home is one of the best advantages that someone who is looking to workout without going to the gym can have. If you've ever found yourself lugging laundry up and down a flight of stairs throughout the day, you can probably relate to this idea.

It gets tiring. For this exercise, begin by standing at the bottom of your stairs. Put one foot on the first step, with the other foot standing on the floor that is underneath of the first step. Shift your weight into the foot that is on the stairs and then lift your other knee up to hip height.

If you want to make this workout even harder, there are a few options. One of them is to instead of standing on the first step, you stand on the second step and then pull your opposite knee to hip height.

This will force you to use more energy in order to come up to stand on the second step. The other option is to twist the body to the left and to the right once you have come up to stand with your knee raised on the step.

Keeping the hips as still as possible, twist to each side before stepping back to the ground. You should complete this exercise on each leg at least 15 times on each side, and repeat on each leg three times. This should not take you more than ten minutes to complete.

At-Home Workout 2: Running the Stairs

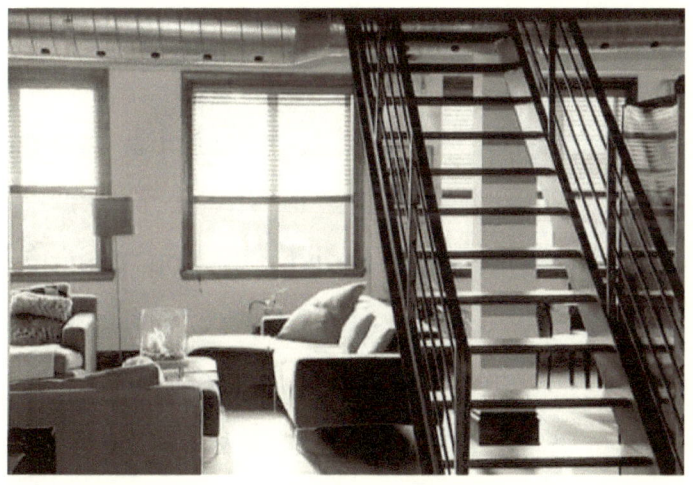

If you're looking for more cardio instead of toning, a great way to accomplish this inside of the home is to partake in running the stairs. Keep in mind, even for someone who is in good shape, running the stairs can prove to be difficult.

For this exercise, you can start at either the bottom or the top of your set of stairs, although it is probably better to start at the bottom of the stairs so that you're getting more resistance as you climb upwards instead of run downwards.

Run up and down the stairs five times each way. Go as fast as you can. Make sure that you have a stopwatch at your disposal, so you can take thirty second breaks when the going gets tough. Did you know that sprinting burns more calories than does jogging?

When you sprint, your body is able to metabolize faster, and this results in weight loss. This is why sprinting up and down the stairs is recommended. If you practice enough, you'll be able to get to a point where you can do more than ten stairs runs in a ten minute window.

At-Home Workout 3: Spider Lunges

In addition to using the stairs, you can also simply use your living room floor. For spider lunges, what you want to do is start in a plank position. From plank, keeping the torso as still and as straight as possible, pick up your right leg and bring it to the outside of your right hand.

Do not place the foot down on the ground once it's outside of the right hand, let it hover in the air. From here, push the right foot back and place it on the ground so that you're resuming a plank position. Then, do this on the left side. Alternate between both feet for between 12 to 15 reps on each side. Your thighs and your hamstrings will be bumping after this workout.

At-Home Workout 4: Jump Lunges

You should perform jump lunges either right before or right after you perform spider lunges. For this workout, you're going to want to in a lunge position with one of your knees bent at a ninety-degree angle with the knee and the ankle aligned with one another.

Once you sink your hips to complete one lunge, jump so that the opposite leg moves to the lunge position and the leg that was just lunging is now behind you. Sink the hips down so that they are at a ninety-degree angle on the opposite side. Alternate between legs for sixteen repetitions on each side, taking a break when you need to. For this exercise, the arms should be working with the opposite leg that is in the lunge position.

For example, if your right leg is in the lunge position, your left elbow should be bent and your left hand should be in a fist position. This will help you to remain stable when you jump to the other leg.

At-Home Workout 5: Walkouts

You will need a stopwatch or a clock in order to properly perform a walkout routine. Start this exercise by starting your stopwatch and doing ten pushups. Make sure that these are quality pushups.

Next, stand up and do jumping jacks until your stopwatch reads one minute. Afterwards, perform walkouts. Standing up, fold foward and then walk your hands out in front of you until you find yourself in a plank position.

From here, count for five and then begin walking your hands back towards your feet. All of these exercises should be done in a set of ten. This workout is more of a circuit rather than one routine. Take breaks as need be.

At-Home Workout 6: 100 Burpees with a Jump

This next exercise is definately one that you'll probably need to work towards. Essentially, a burpee is a plank and a pushup done one after the other. You will start by standing up.

Next, fold forward and jump your legs back to find yourself in a plank position. Once you're in a plank, do one pushup. When you're in a plank once again after completing your pushup, jump your feet towards your hands, and then jump up so that both of your feet are in the air. This circuit counts as one burpee with a jump. Repeat this one hundred times, and be sure to time yourself as you do this. Seeing your progress will provide you with the motivation that you need to keep repeating this workout over a long period of time.

If you stick with it, you'll eventually be able to upgrade this workout to do two pushups instead of one. From personal experience, it is going to be difficult to get through one hundred burpees when you're first starting out, but the satisfaction that comes with eventually being able to do them is well worth the work and sweat that's involved when you're first starting out. You want to be stronger, right? Burpees are a fabulous way to achieve exactly that.

Chapter 3: An Ab Circuit Guaranteed to Give You a Six Pack

If you're going to be targeting different areas of the body each day, then you're going to need a variety of workouts to choose from for each body part. The following circuit can be implemented on your ab day. You can perform these ab workouts at home, because most of them require laying on the ground:

Ab Workout 1: Suitcases

Begin by laying on your back. Bring your arms up and over your head so that you look like one long pencil. Then, using mostly your core, bend your knees and begin to come up to sit, bringing your arms up and over head. Do not let your feet touch the ground.

Once you're sitting in a curled position, begin to lie back, coming into a pencil position one the ground once again. Repeat this for at least twenty-five repetitions. If you need more resistance, consider holding a weight in your hands and bringing that over your head.

Ab Workout 2: Russian Twists

For this exercise, you're going to want to find a sitting position. With your knees bent, the feet should not be touching the ground. You are hovering your knees in the air. Next, bring both of your hands off to the right side, trying to get both of your hands to touch the ground on the outside of your right knee.

Once you've touched the ground with your hands on the right side, bring the hands back to center before moving the hands off to the left side. Repeat this with your knees in towards your chest and without the feet touching the ground for twenty-five repetitions on each side. If you can't do fifty repetitions in a row, bring the toes to the floor, but resist the urge to bring all of the weight in your feet back down to the ground.

Ab Workout 3: Leg Lifts

This ab workout will help to target your lower abs. Lay down and put both of your feet in the air. Once your feet are in the air, begin to lower both of them at the same time until they are hovering about six inches from the ground. Once they're hovering here, pause for between three to five seconds, before lifting the legs back up into the air using your core strength.

A pro tip for this exercise is to pull your stomach in so that you can make your lower abs as flat as possible. Otherwise, you will not see the greatest level of benefits from this workout.

Ab Workout 4: Leg Reaches

For this workout, you should also be laying on your back

with both of your legs in the air. Reach your arms up and towards your toes, using your core strength to touch your toes with your fingertips.

If you can't touch your fingertips to your toes, just try to get to them as close as you can. Again, you want to make sure that your stomach is flat and that all fat is pulling in towards the abdomen in order for this exercise to really work. Repeat this exercise at least twenty-five times, if not more.

Ab Workout 5: Side Planks

This workout will target the sides of your abs, rather than the front of your abs. Begin to rolling off to one side of your body, either the right or the left. From here, bring either your forearm or your hand to the ground and lift your body up so that the only parts of your body that are touching the ground are the one hand and one foot. Stack the hips on top of one another, and reach the hand that is closest to the ceiling up into the air.

Hold this position for between thirty seconds to one minute, before switching sides. If you lift the hips up and down as you're in a side plank, you'll feel even more intensity.

Chapter 4: Three Back Exercises that Require No Equipment

No one likes to have a flabby back, especially during bikini season. The workouts below will target key areas of the back that will chisel your back to be the best looking thing on the beach.

Back Workout 1: Fire Hydrants

If you've ever seen a dog urinating on a fire hydrant, then you can see how this workout gets its name. Come onto your hands and knees so that the back and spine are flat. With your spine straight, use only your back muscles to lift the right leg up with the knee still bent.

When you bring the knee back down, don't let it touch the ground. Repeat this on each side at least fifteen times, or until you can feel your lower back muscles straining.

Back Workout 2: Alternating Donkey Kicks

This workout also targets the lower back, and many people use fire hydrants in conjunction with alternative donkey kicks. Begin with your hands and knees in a table top position. From here, lift one knee off of the ground and pull it towards your chest. Then, send the knee back until the leg is straight, trying to keep the torso as still as possible. Continue this as well for at least fifteen reps.

Back Workout 3: Butterflies

For this workout, you can stand. Bring your hands by your ears so that the elbows are bent, and bend over so that your back is flat. Next, lift the elbows away from the ears, making sure that the shoulder blades are pushing towards one another. Repeat this exercise for at least thirty reps, because of the fact that you will not be using weights. If you want to experience more intensity, using weights for this exercise will certainly intensify the workout.

Chapter 5: Understanding the Muscles of the Body

If we were to discuss literally all of the muscles on the human body, it's safe to say that we would take up all of the pages in this book and then some. Instead of discussing all of the body's muscles, this chapter is going to talk about all of the muscles in the body that can be targeted when working out.

We will start at the top of the head and work our way down to the lower half of the body. Each of these muscle groups can be targeted through precise exercises that will strengthen each group in a unique way.

If you know the muscles that you want to target, you'll be able to do workouts that are specific, efficient, and detailed. Let's take a look at what these muscle groups are and how you can begin to strengthen them in the appropriate ways.

Major Muscles Found at the Neck

There are two major muscles that you can work out that can be found around the neck region of the body. These are the upper trapezius and the levator scapulae.

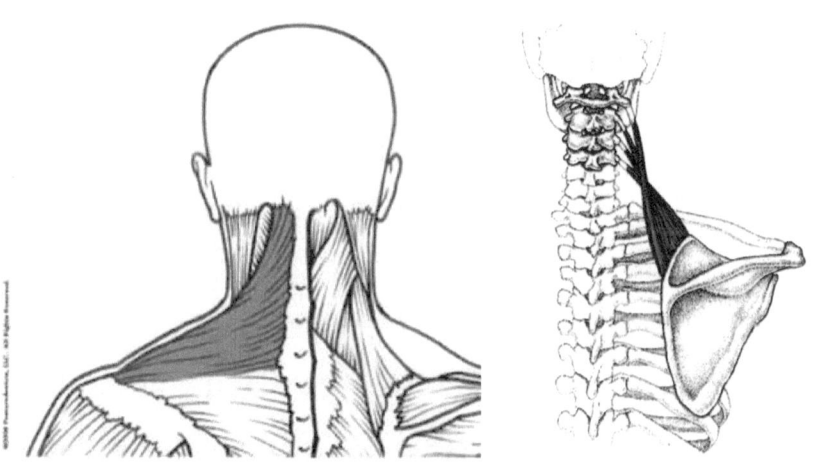

The photo on the left depicts the upper trapezius, while the photo on the left illustrates the position of the levator scapulae. The upper trapezius is connected to the trapezius muscle group of fibers that actually extends in a trapezoidal-like shape all the way to the midpoint on the back. There's a chance that you have already heard of this muscle group, as this area of the body is commonly referred to as the "traps" or in this case, the "upper traps". Within the physical therapy world, there is a clear tendency to blame this muscle group for being tight and tense.

You may already notice this while you're sitting at your office desk or when you wake up in the morning. Often, people are advised that the remedy for alleviating the tension felt within this area towards the base of the neck is to stretch and massage it. While yes, this does feel good in the short-term, in the long-term this stretching and massaging does not do much to make a real difference in how you're going to feel. The reality is that if you want the upper trapezius muscles to feel less tense, then you should be trying to strengthen them.

While the trapezius muscle is largely part of an entire muscles group, the group of fibers that comprise the levator scapulae are mostly responsible for holding the scapula (popularly known as the shoulder blades) in place on the body and also lifting the shoulders when this action is necessary.

Needless to say, if you're going to be lifting weights, you want to make sure that your levator scapulae is strong and intact. When the levator scapulae is stiff, you may feel unable to turn your head from side to side easily. Another common problem that people with weak levator scapulae experience and complain of includes a shortness of breath when this muscle is twisted. Some people describe this as feeling as if they are going to have a panic attack.

A great exercise that can help to strengthen both the upper trapezius and the levator scapulac are shoulder shrugs. There's a chance that you have already done shoulder shrugs in your life at one time or another, and they are a great way to specifically target the upper back region on which you're trying to concentrate your energy.

What's more, you can easily do this workout at your office or at home while you're watching your kids or even when you're watching television. The first step in this exercise is to make sure that you're standing with good posture. The next step is to raise your shoulders as high as they can go (preferably near your ears if you can get your shoulders there). After that, count to two in your head before bringing your shoulders back down the back, making sure to keep the shoulders plugged into one another as you complete this movement. Repeat this exercise at least twenty times.

If you're sitting here thinking that you are not going to feel any type of strength by doing this exercise without weights, you may be surprised to find that you will actually feel your muscles strengthening after doing this; however, over time it's safe to say that you will probably need more weight added in order to keep improving.

Since this book promotes the use of free workout methods, instead of jumping to the conclusion that you need to buy a set of weights, perhaps instead grab two of your heaviest books and hold these in your hands as you do the shoulder shrugs. This way, your upper back and neck muscles are responsible for more weight. And remember, your neck is relatively delicate when compared to the rest of your body. Don't overdo it.

Muscles Found in the Core

As we move down the length of the torso, the next part of the body that we're going to discuss is the core. It may come as a surprise to you, but the core works during pretty much every movement that we make.

I have heard it said that the key to becoming stronger and more balanced during any workout or sport is to develop a stable core because of the fact that the core is so crucial in almost every movement that is possible for the human body. Let's take a look at some of the key muscles that exist within the core itself:

1. **The Transverse Abdominals**
2. **The Multifidus**
3. **The Diaphragm**
4. **The Pelvic Floor**

The Transverse Abdominals

You will also sometimes see the transverse abdominals referred to as the transverse abdominis. This is the deepest layer of the core, and they play a huge role in not only protecting a large portion of the torso but also help to stabilize the spine. The transverse abdominal is located underneath of the common "six-pack" abs that we closely associate with the core.

It's important to note that this muscle group is activated almost whenever a part of the body moves. It should be obvious how important the transverse abdominals are.

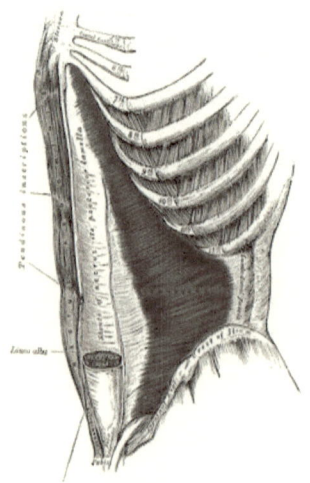

Some great workouts that are free and target the deep transverse abdominal muscles include the plank, and the glute lift. The exercise with which you are probably most familiar is the plank. A plank can be done by lying down on your belly and placing either your forearms or your hands directly underneath of your shoulders.

Pushing down, you lift the rest of the body up into the air so that you resemble a piece of wood; everything is flat and even on the body.

There is no curvature, and no part of the body is more elevated than another. Hold this position for between thirty to sixty seconds, and I can almost guarantee that you're going to feel some sort of strengthening in the core. Generally speaking, it's more challenging on the shoulders to do the plank on your hands, while doing the plank on your forearms will alleviate some of the sensation that you're going to feel in the shoulders. You can also partake in side planking to strengthen the sides of the transverse abdominals.

The other type of exercise that is great for improving the transverse abdominis is known as the glute lift. Begin by coming onto your hands and knees. With your hands firmly pressing into the ground, lift one leg up so that the bottom of your foot is facing towards the ceiling. There should be a bend in your knee.

Once the foot is pressing towards the ceiling, begin to make micromovements with the leg, lifting up the leg so that you feel action taking place in the glute. Repeat this exercise for between fifteen to thirty reps, and then switch to the other leg.

It may not seem like this would be an exercise for the core but rather for the glute, but when you're in this position you are using a lot of core energy to keep the leg lifted. In a way, you will be strengthening both the core and the glutes simultaneously.

The Multifidus

This is one of the smaller muscles that exist along the spine, but don't let its size full you. The multifidus is one of the most important muscle groups that exist along the spine as well as one of the strongest.

This group of muscles helps to keep the spine straight and distributes our body weight so that we can function properly. Below is a picture of the multifidus muscle along the spine:

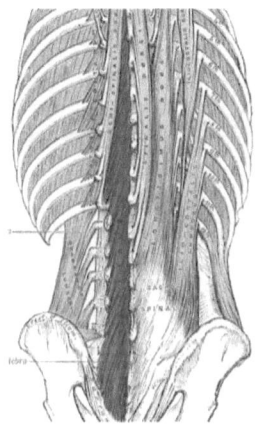

Without the capabilities that the multifidus muscle group allows, you would not be able to perform many of the functions that you may currently take for granted such as bending backwards, to one side or the other, and even turning onto our sides when we go to sleep.

One of the most prevalent problems that people have that deals with the multifidus is lower back pain. There is a specific multifidus exercise that can help to strengthen the lower multifidus and prevent this type of injury. It's known as the leg lift. To perform this exercise, begin by lying on your back. Bend one knee and bring your foot to the floor.

The other leg will be straight out in front of you. Again, using micromovements begin to lift the leg to about the height of your core, and then lower it back down but do not allow the leg to touch the floor. Do this for about twenty-five reps on each leg.

Once you have become comfortable with this exercise, you can expand it by perhaps tracing the alphabet with this leg, or performing leg circles.

The Diaphragm
The diaphragm, whether you knew it or not, is in fact a muscle. Located within the torso, the abdomen muscles

protect this muscle so that it can in turn protect the chest and the organs within it.

This muscle is what allows us to breathe, so it's obviously important to have this muscle be strong, especially if you're looking to develop and maintain an overall healthy lifestyle.

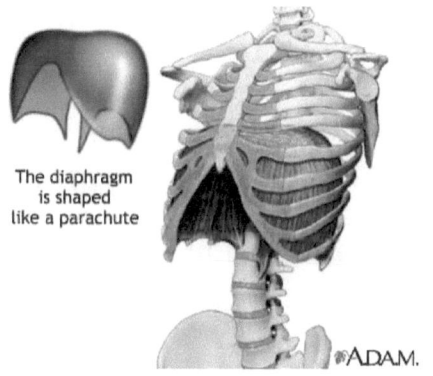

The diaphragm is shaped like a parachute

Many singers will use breathing exercises to strengthen the diaphragm so that they will be more successful in their singer endeavors. This may sound funny, but one of these exercises includes blowing up a balloon. It's safe to say that nearly everyone has blown up a balloon at some point in their life. Of course, blowing up a balloon is technically not a free exercise, but it is a relatively cheap one.

What's more, if you're at work when you perform this exercise, you can attach a string to your balloon once you're finished with it and give it to a coworker to brighten their day.

The Pelvic Floor

The last portion of the core is the pelvic floor. The pelvic floor is a muscle that supports and protects the bladder and bowel region, as well as the uterus region in women. Obviously, as you get older, it's important that you keep this organ group protected and intact. A great exercise that is often used to make the pelvic floor stronger is known as the bridge. This is also a pose that it often used in yoga frequently (which is the subject of the next chapter). In bridge, lay on your back with your palms facing down. You'll want your hands to be by your hips. The knees are bent. Once you find yourself in this position, the next step is to lift the lower, middle and then upper back up and off of the ground.

You'll want to really push the hips and the pelvis high so that they're reaching towards the ceiling. You'll also want to press down with your feet quite a bit. Over time, this will help to provide your pelvis with more stability and strength.

Your Quadricep Muscles

The last muscle group at which we're going to look are the quads. The quads are largely located in your thigh region and are comprised of four large muscles. These muscles are:

1. **The Rectus Femoris**
2. **The Vastus Lateralis**
3. **The Vastus Medialis**
4. **The Vastus Intermedius**

The picture below should provide you with information on where each of these fine muscles are located:

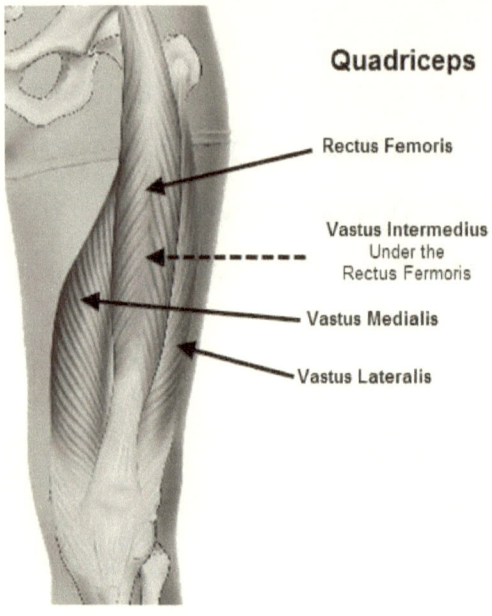

One of the best workouts that you can do for all of the muscles in your quads are squats. Of course, doing squats would be even more beneficial to you if you were to go to a gym and use weights to accomplish this goal, but if you're first starting out or you are looking to save money by avoiding the gym, then doing squats in your home is the next best thing.

It's important to note that you can definately still see results by implementing these strategies. Begin by standing up straight, and then lift one foot and bring it to a ninety-degree angle in front of you, making sure that the ankle is in line with the knee.

Begin to bend down, so that your back is completely straight and your back knee is almost touching the floor, but not quite.

Once you're down here, begin to lift yourself back up, making sure to notice the strength that you're using in both your legs and your core. Repeat this one each leg for between twelve to sixteen times. You're sure to see fast results if you take on this challenge on a tri-weekly basis.

Chapter 6: Yoga ~ How to Do a Sun Salutation

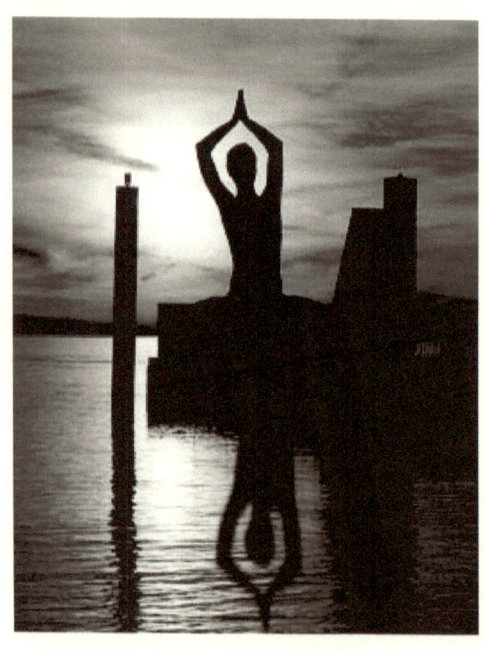

The next chapter on which we're going to focus our attention is one that is both good for the body as well as the mind. Yes, we are going to be talking about the topic of yoga. As a physical practice, yoga can offer many benefits, and one of the best aspects of yoga as a physical practice is that there are variations of each pose that anyone can do.

This means that yoga is for young people just as much as it is for older people. It's can be equally beneficial to someone who is overweight as well as someone who is extremely fit and looking to find new ways to experiment with their strength and flexibility. This chapter is going to focus on how to do a basic sun salutation.

Sun salutations require strength as well as flexibility, so it can provide you with the ability to get stronger and stretch both at the same time. Many people do sun salutations in the morning so that their body can wake up more easily. We will also talk about the breath, which is an essential part of any good yoga practice.

The Breath

We have all seen photos of people doing fancy yoga poses in their fancy yoga clothes. These pictures and these people depicts the idea that these people have everything in their lives together. They appear peaceful and calm, and they

seemingly have nothing to worry about at all. While these pictures are pretty, they don't really represent what yoga is all about. Yoga, at is core, is about the breath. It's not about getting to a point where you can put both legs behind your head (although, that is cool, admittedly). Arguably the most popular type of yoga these days in the United States is vinyasa yoga.

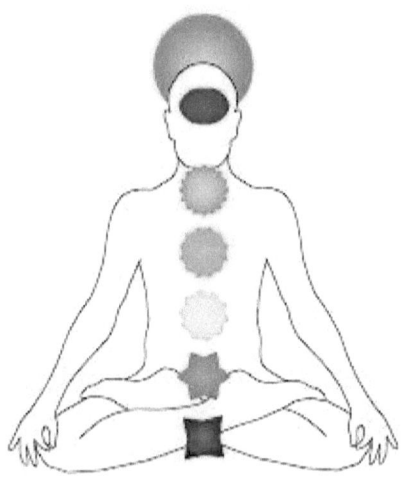

This is a type of yoga that is based in poses that link or flow together via pose sequencing. In vinyasa yoga, your primary goal is to link every movement that you're making with your breath.

There are essentially only two ways that you are breathing during any given activity, regardless of what it is; you're either inhaling or you're exhaling. In this way, yoga can provide an individual with the opportunity to move with the body and find relaxation through linking the various yoga poses with one another.

An additional aspect of yoga is the idea that while you are doing these various poses, you should *only* be thinking about these specific movements. When you think in the present moment, with intention and move in conjunction with the breath, you can discover more of your body through the avenue that yoga provides. Yoga begins with the breath.

A Sun Salutation

Arguably the most foundational sequences to a vinyasa yoga class is known as a sun salutation. If you ever decide to go to a yoga studio and learn from a certified yoga instructor, it's safe to say that you will do some form of a sun salutation during class at some point. In Sanskrit, a sun salutation is known as a *Surya Namaskar*. The primary reasoning behind partaking in this sequence of poses is so that the body can properly warm up. That's why this sequence is usually done during the beginning of class.

It's best to do a sun salutation during the beginning of class and on an empty stomach. Another great reason why sun salutations are highly encouraged in yoga is because they call the individual to give gratitude towards the sun and more broadly all of what makes life possible.

Sometimes it can be easy to forget about all of the forces that come together that make life happen each and every day.

Sequencing a Surya Namaskar

Here we will take a look at the basic structure of a sun salutation. After learning this sequence, you'll have a better understanding of not only what a sun salutation is, but also how to do the foundational poses that are often found in a yoga class. Of course, a sun salutation is only the starting block.

There are so many other wonderful poses that yoga can offer you. The best thing about yoga is that you don't necessarily have to pay for it these days. Yoga classes typically run between thirteen to fifteen dollars per class, and I have even seen them priced as high as eighteen dollars for one hour!

If you have access to YouTube, you can become just as skilled at yoga as someone who goes to class once a week, and you don't even have to leave your living room. Let's take a look at the poses that make up a sun salutation. Please note that the pose name will first appear in Sanskrit and then in English.

Pose 1: Tadasana

The first pose of the sun salutation is known as mountain pose, or Tadasana in Sanskrit. Mountain pose is the most foundational pose that's found in yoga. The basic idea surrounding mountain pose is that even when you're doing a fancy arm balance or a handstand, you are always supposed to feel as strong as you do in mountain pose.

This pose itself it quite simple. You stand with both of your feet on the ground at the top of your mat. Your hands should be by your side, with your palms facing away from you.

Sometimes, one of the most difficult aspects of this pose can be the idea that your shoulders should be down your back and plugged in towards one another. When you're positioned in this manner, think about closing the eyes, and looking inward. This is typically cued as an "exhale" position" throughout a vinyasa yoga practice.

Pose 2: Urdhva Hastasana

Technically, this pose is referred to as, "upward hands pose" pose, so it may just be easier for you to refer to it as urdhva hastasana. After your hands are by your sides, you raise them over your head.

Some people think of this part as the actual "saluting" of the sun during a sun salutation. The arms go over the head, with the palms facing towards one another. Similar to the Tadasana position, the shoulders remain down the back and plugged into one another. In contrast to Tadasana, Urdhva Hastasana is typically done during an inhale.

Pose 3: Uttanasana

After your arms are over your head in urdhva hastasana, the next pose is known as "uttanasana" or forward fold. Often, people will bring their hands from overhead through their heart's center so that the palms touch, before they hinge at the hips and fold forward. Ideally, the legs will be completely straight in this position and the hands will be touching the floor; however, it is easy to guess that not everyone is this flexible.

For a beginner, bending the knees so that the belly can rest on the thighs is completely acceptable. This way, the pose is more accessible.

Uttanasana is done during an exhale within the sun salutation.

Pose 4: Lifting the Gaze, Lengthening the Spine

Truth be told, there isn't really a Sanskrit term for this next pose; in fact, it should not truly be considered a pose but rather a transition to the next actual pose. The instructor at this point will typically say something along the lines of, "lift the gaze, lengthen the spine long", and this generally comes after the forward fold position in which you find yourself.

Pose 5: Chaturunga Dandasana

In English, Chaturunga Dandasana can be translated to mean "four-limbed staff pose". After you've lifted the gaze, found a flat back and have lengthened your spine, the next step in the sun salutation is to shoot your legs back into a plank-like position and bend the elbows so that you're in a low push up.

Remember, the goal is to seem as calm and steady as you felt in Tadasana. In this low pushup, the gaze should be slightly lifted. The pelvis should be slightly tucked just like it is in Tadasana, and the back should be perfectly straight. Pushing down into your low pushup is an exhale motion.

Pose 6: Urdhva Mukha Svanasana

The next pose in the sequence is known in English as "Upward-Facing Dog" pose. After moving into your low pushup, you will begin to straighten your arms into this position on the inhale. Bringing the tops of your toes to the floor so that they're pressing down, this is the essence of the pose. This is done on an inhalation.

Pose 7: Adho Mukha Svanasana

Finally, we have gotten to the pose that perhaps everyone largely associates with yoga. Downward facing dog is performed on the exhale following the inhale from upward facing dog. Instead of having the hips and pelvis bent towards the floor, the hips rise up so that your seat is high in the air. The shoulders are away from the ears, and both hands are pressing down towards the floor.

This is meant to be a restorative pose, and it's safe to say when you're first starting your yoga practice, you're going to need some restoration in your practice. If you still with the practice, you will be able to easily hang out in downward facing dog for a long period of time; however, when you're first starting out this may prove to be a bit difficult (depending on what your strength level is).

Since we've already gone over the rest of the poses in detail, the following poses complete the sun salutation sequence. Remember to do the poses in this order, or else they won't make sense for your body:

Pose 8: Uttanasana

Pose 9: Urdhva Hastasana

Pose 10: Tadasana

Those are the basic poses that comprise the sun salutation. Of course, since you are reading this book because you want to be exposed to workouts that can be done without having to spend any money, one of the best ways to utilize the sun salutation is when you first get up in the morning. If you do between five to seven sun salutations each morning, not only will you wake up more easily, but you'll also be able to develop your yoga practice over time. The tips in this book regarding the sun salutations can help you to figure out the intricacies of each yoga pose within the sun salutation, while looking up basic yoga poses on YouTube can also provide you with information that you may not yet know.

Don't be afraid to experiment with the body, and as you dive deeper into your yoga practice try to keep in mind that fear can really get in the way if you let it. Remember, you are stronger than you think. Your body can do truly amazing things if you let it.

Chapter 7: Meditation, Mindfulness, and Breathing

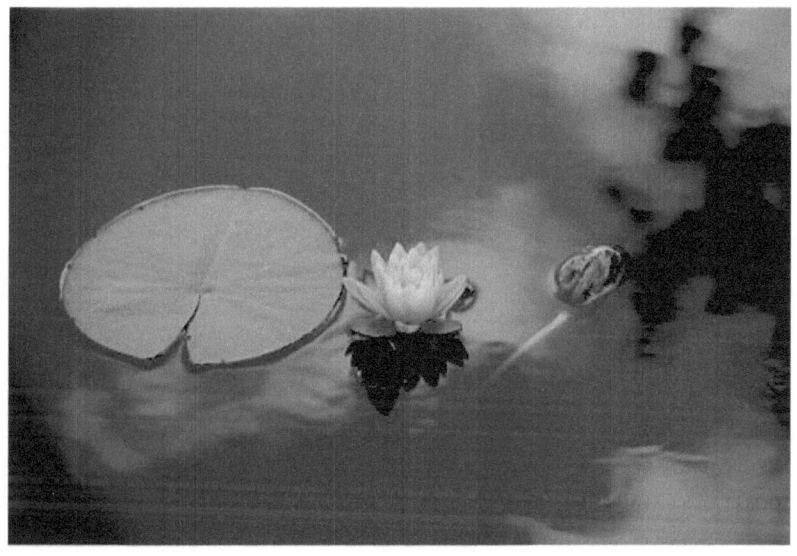

While we already discussed some of the importance of mindful breathing in the previous chapter regarding yoga, this chapter is going to dig even deeper into this topic. While yoga can often be associated with meditation and an overall lifestyle that supports mindfulness, the two can also be distinct from one another.

This chapter will explore what meditation is, how to do it, and will also provide you with some tips on how to lead a more mindful lifestyle.

What is Meditation and How Do I Do It?

Meditation, in its most basic sense, is the activity of sitting still and taking some time to clear the mind.

When you meditate, the goal is not to think about a single thing obsessively; rather, it is to resist the urge to focus on anything that is related to the minutiae of your everyday life.

Overtime, the goal of anyone who has a consistent and serious meditation practice is to find a deeper sense of what reality truly is. Again, it must be reiterated that this does not mean a deeper sense of how you're going to make more money or how you're going to get more recognition on social media. Meditation goes deeper than that. When an individual meditates, he or she hopes to transform his or her emotional habits and patterns.

If you meditate often enough, you will soon be able to see the reasons behind your anger, or your sadness, or your fear more easily than before. What's more, when you encounter these types of situations that make you angry or sad or scared in your everyday life, you will be better equipped to handle them because of your ability to recognize your triggers in the first place. I know this might sound strange, but meditation can be truly transformative if you're open to it. Trust me, I've been developing a meditation practice for quite some time now.

How to Properly Meditate

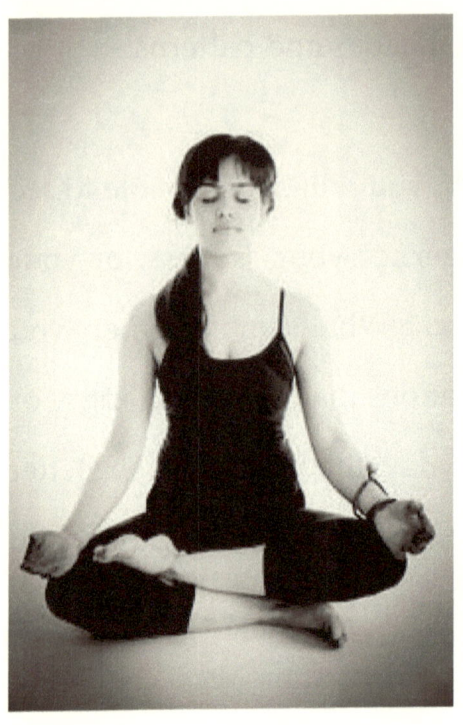

One of the first things to think about when you're going to start practicing meditation is how to find a comfortable position with the body. When you're first starting out, this usually means that you're going to want to be sitting in a chair. If you're in relatively good shape and know that you can sustain a good posture for a certain period of time, you might consider using a cushion on the floor instead of a chair.

A chair with a sturdy back should be used when people are experiencing bad posture or know that they can't sit upright for longer periods of time. A cushion on the other hand, requires that you find good posture before you start meditating.

Another great option for meditation is to put a yoga block underneath of your seat so that your tush is slightly more elevated than your knees.

In this position with your legs crossed and your knees angled towards the floor, you have found yourself a good meditation seat.

How to Enter into a Meditation Space

After you've found your seat in whichever way feels most comfortable to you, the next step is to enter into your meditation space. There are various ways that this can be done, and the way that you choose to do this depends on a couple of different factors. If you're an incredibly spiritual person and are looking to dive deeper into your religious or spiritual self, you might begin your meditation by chanting a particular mantra.

These mantras vary widely in their meaning, but what you are basically doing when you chant a mantra is calling into your awareness a particular Hindu god or goddess. Again, the intricacies of each god and goddess who play a part in making yoga and meditation what it truly is are beyond the scope of this book; however, if you are interested in chanting prior to beginning a meditation practice, these different deities are definitely aspects of the Hindu culture into which you should look.

It's safe to say that chanting is one of the more serious ways to get into your meditation space. There are other ways that you can do it, and these ways are considered to be less extreme. For example, if you are not confident about chanting yet and would prefer something more mainstream, maybe start with an OM instead.

There is a chance that you've heard of the OM before. OM is also a mantra, but one that contains less in terms of Hindu language attached to it. OM was first seen in what is known as the *Upanishads*, which is a group of sacred Hindu texts.

The beauty of the sound OM is that it can be interpreted in a variety of different ways. For example, some people interpret OM as being the sound of universal peace.

Others see it as being a sound that resonates universal energy, and still others see OM as being reflective of the idea that all people are connected through peace in some way. Others see OM as being an interpretation of all of these different types of ideas. In this way, OM is everything.

Some people, while they want to be able to reap the

benefits of a sound and relaxing meditation practice, have problems associating anything concretely religious to it. For example, many people who are practicing Catholics or practice another Western religion devoutly do not really want to be chanting in another language, even if "OM" does not actually mean anything inherently religious. If you find yourself within this category of people, you're certainly not alone, and there are still options available to you.

Instead of chanting anything before you sink into your meditation space, you can simply sit still, close your eyes, and begin to breathe. After you've started to breathe, you can inhale and think to yourself, "Let". On your exhale, you can think to yourself, "Go". This mantra, "Let Go" is something that does not need to be religious or spiritual in nature. You can associate your meditation with your breathing. It's as simple as that.

Guided Meditation

Maybe you have heard about people who are able to meditate for forty-five minutes without taking a break, and maybe you have not. These people do exist, but they didn't become able to perform this type of meditation overnight.

Meditating for long periods of time begins with meditating for small periods of time. When you're first starting out, you're going to want to try and meditate every single day. Yes, that's right. Daily. This may seem like a lot or a little to you, but it only takes five minutes per day. I'll be honest, as someone who does try to meditate on a consistent basis, I must admit that there are some days where I really don't want to look inward.

Maybe I'm busy, or maybe there is something going on with me emotionally that I am afraid to look in the face and contemplate. Whatever the case may be, the reality is that there are going to be days when you just can't seem to

68

conjure the energy to meditate. What's important is that even if you don't make it the entire five minutes that you should allot yourself per day, you still need to make the attempt. Sit down in a quiet place. Attempt to concentrate. See what happens. If you fail, there is always tomorrow.

In addition to making the attempt, you should also resist the urge to be too hard on yourself. If you are too hard on yourself, there will come a day when you just give up and stop meditating altogether.

While meditating for five minutes may not seem like much in writing, the reality is that sometimes five minutes can sometimes feel like it's as long as an hour of your time. A great way to initiate yourself with what meditation can offer you is to participate in what's known as guided meditation.

Guided meditation is exactly what it sounds like; however, if you don't want to spend money on someone who can physically be with you as a guide during meditation, the next best thing is to install an application onto your phone. This application is free and it's called Headspace. Of course, they prompt you to also upgrade to experience everything that their application has to offer, but there is plenty to do on the application without every purchasing a thing.

With Headspace, there are ten levels of meditation, and each one becomes a bit longer than the next. There is more actual silence during the later sessions of meditation, while the earlier ones include more of a satisfying voice dictated by a British man. You have nothing to lose by trying Headspace; and no, this isn't some sort of plug for the application. I have used Headspace in my own life and have definitely found it to be quite useful.

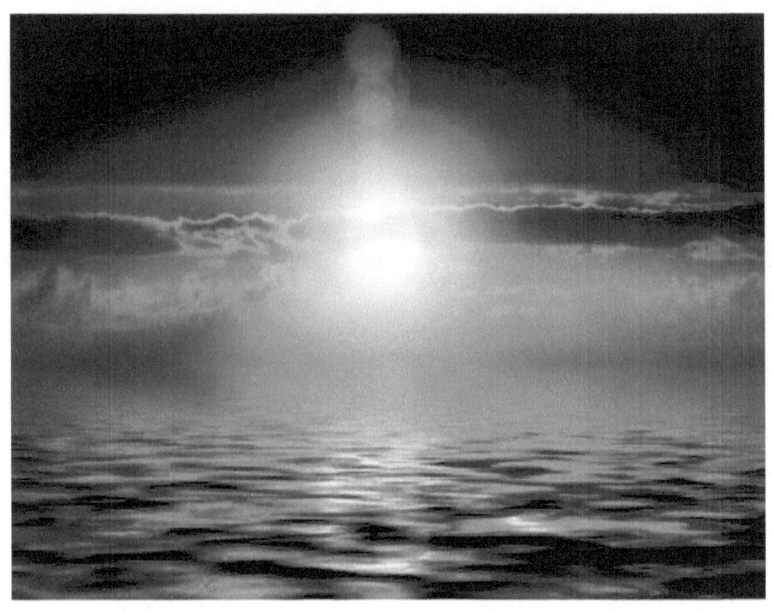

Chapter 8: Why Stretching is as Important as Exercising

Many people are under the impression that stretching is not *that* important a component to a workout regime. Most people are prone to thinking that they can get by only stretching when they have the time; otherwise, forget it. This chapter is going to primarily look at the reasons why stretching is important and why you should refuse to miss it when working out.

While stretching may not be the most popular thing to do, taking the time to do it properly can be the difference between being able to keep up with your workout regime over the long-term. Imagine if you were to pull a muscle or worse tear something because you did not take the time that you needed to stretch. Not only would you be upset about it in the short-term, but it would also negatively influence your performance for years to come.

The Benefits of Stretching

Stretching should be done on a daily basis. This means that even if you're someone who is generally against working out to an extreme form, you can still benefit from integrating stretching into your life.

Once you start stretching on a daily basis, one of the first results that you're going to see is...well, more flexibility obviously. Having more flexibility allows the body to move more easily, and who doesn't want that? Let's take a look at some of the other benefits stretching can offer.

1. Greater Blood Flow

Some people decide to stretch every morning because stretching delivers more blood to the entire body. This helps to awaken the body, and therefore will help you to need one less shot of espresso to make it through the day. This increase in blood flow includes blood flow to the brain. By stretching in the morning, you'll be able to think with more clarity and get through the day with more ease.

2. Greater Stability on Your Feet

When you take the time to stretch, you are also taking the time to increase your ability to balance. This is especially important as you get older, because as your age increases you are less able to physically react fast enough when something gets in your way. Stretching provides the body with a better sense of itself, and this in turn allows an individual to finely tune their balance.

3. Generally Less Pain

One of the many reasons why yoga has become so popular in recent years is because of its ability to alleviate pain. No one wants to take pain medication on a regular basis if it can be helped, and with the pharmaceutical craze that has swept the United States up within the last decade, it's safe to say that your physician may try to medicate you *before* they advise you to simply stretch it out. The home remedy is also much less expensive than the over-the-counter one.

4. Deeper Exercises

If you're looking to increase your flexibility as well as exercise in conjunction with this, then another reason why you should be participating in both exercising and stretching at the same time is because becoming more flexible will help you to deepen your exercise regime.

Think about it. If you are trying to constantly improve

your body as well as your mind, this means taking it to new positions and levels of endurance. When you stretch, your body is more easily able to take on tasks that you have set for yourself. For example, if you decide to do a set of squats – what is the point in doing the squats if you are not going to squat down to a full ninety-degree angle? If you are only able to do something haphazardly because of your flexibility, you will never be able to get the full expression of the exercise down to a science. Thus, the quality of your workout regime will be sacrificed.

5. Less Injuries

This should be fairly obvious, but when you're able to do more with your body in terms of flexibility, you will be less likely to injure yourself in the process. It's generally understood that you should never go out and do any type of exercising before warming up the body even a tiny bit.

When you take the time to stretch prior to doing some sort of straining activity on the body, you are less likely to shock the muscles into harsh movement. This is especially true in the morning. Additionally, dynamic stretching is a great way to get the body moving quickly.

This type of movement includes stretching that is continuous such as arm circles or running in place.

The Different Type of Stretching That's Available to You

Now that you know about the different benefits that stretching can provide to you, let's now briefly take a look at two types of stretching that are quite popular these days. These include dynamic stretching and ballistic stretching.

Dynamic Stretching

Dynamic stretching involves moving as you stretch, with the idea being that you are stretching the muscles that you're going to be using during your workout. For example, lunges are sometimes used in a way that promotes dynamic stretching rather than simply working out, because when you twist while you lunge you are able to warm up muscles that you are going to be using during a sport that you're going to play or a cross fit class that you're going to take. It's widely understood that dynamic stretching can widen your range of motion prior to your workout, and this can deliver great benefits to your overall training goals.

Ballistic Stretching

Ballistic stretching is actually a form of dynamic stretching, but there is less overall movement involved generally. In ballistic stretching, the area of the body that is being stretched is bounced gently so that the body part is pushed past its normal range of motion.

Ballistic stretches are often used in sports such as football, martial arts, basketball, and dance. There is some controversy surrounding how beneficial ballistic stretching can truly be. Some people think that it broadens your range of motion in great ways, while others think that there is a great risk of injury in partaking in ballistic stretching.

Christopher J. Davis, M.D. /Anna G Taylor

Daily stretching Routine

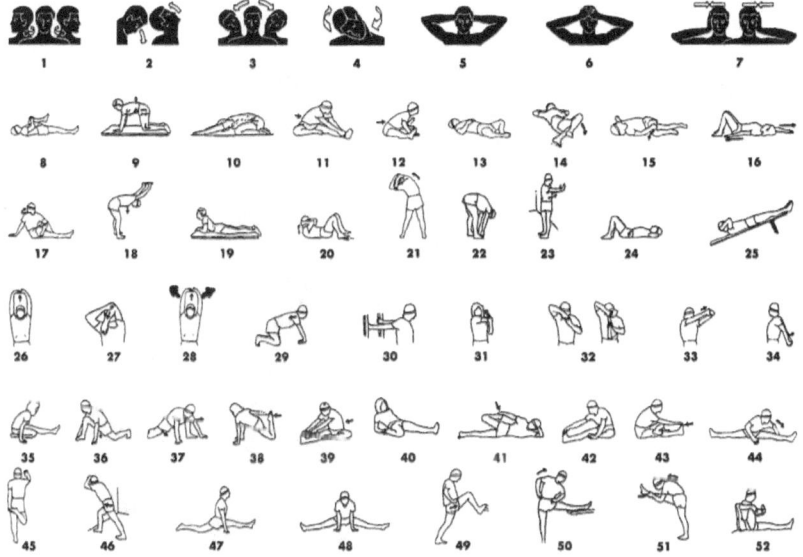

Chapter 9: Developing Healthy Eating Habits

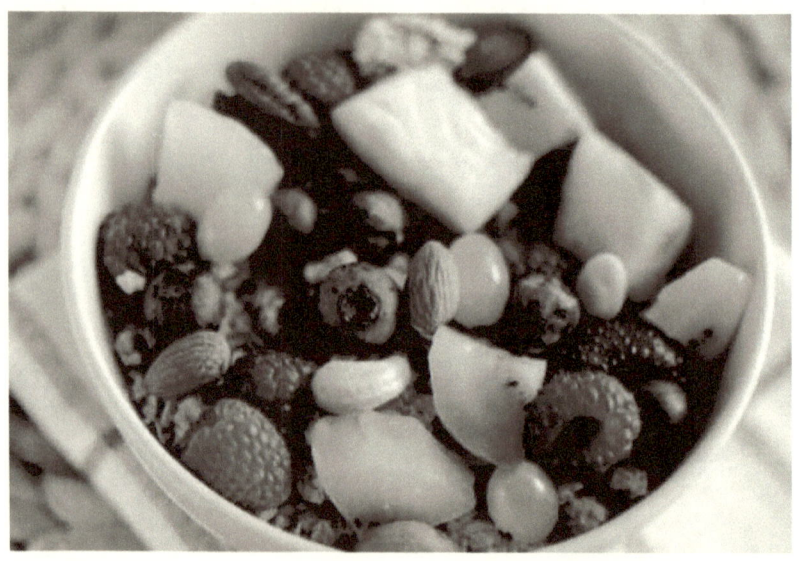

Our conversation about exercising and mindfulness would not be complete without a discussion about healthy and mindful eating as well. This chapter will discuss what you can do to better your eating habits. If you have terrible eating habits now, it's important to first recognize this fact, but also understand that dieting is a task that is best done little-by-little.

No one has lost weight by seeing or expecting results overnight, and this is the primary reason why people give up during the dieting process. Instead of looking at this chapter as a mechanism that will immediately enable you to lose weight, it might be a better idea to look at it as smaller pieces that you can strive for over the long-term. It might be a cliché, but it's also true; if you want to successfully diet, you are going to need to partake in a complete lifestyle change.

If you hate what you're eating and cannot wait for the day when your diet will come to an end, you will most likely resort back to your bad eating habits and gain back all of the weight that you intended to lose. Let's take a look at some of the ways that you can better yourself from a dieting perspective.

Clean(er) Eating

Clean eating refers to the idea that an individual is going to seek out eating foods that are not very processed or handled before being consumed. This means that when you go grocery shopping, you stay away from the chips and cookie aisle.

Instead, you gravitate towards the raw fruits and vegetables, as well as the aisle that holds the nuts, whole grains such as rice, and legumes.

Often times, the food industry as a whole is not heavily regulated (even though the FDA will have you believe otherwise). Some foods that are advertised as being healthy are actually anything but good for you, so it's best to stay away from processed foods altogether when possible.

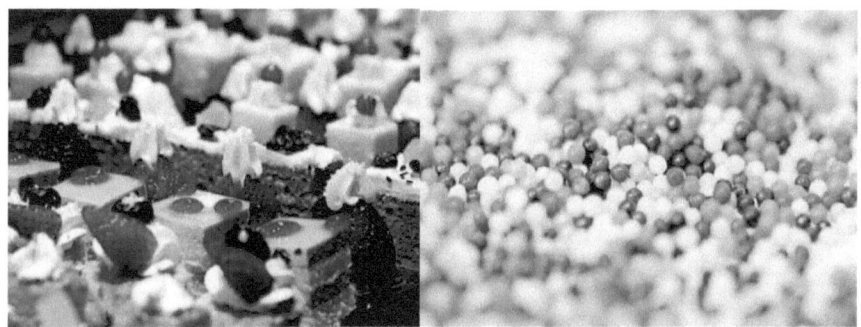

Lastly, sugar is a big reason why processed foods are considered to be "dirty" when compared to the benefits of clean eating. Sugar inevitably turns into fat when digested, so it's best to avoid processed sugars, including the sugar that is found in soda, whenever possible. You may not know this, but a leading factor of obesity in the United States is due to unchecked soda consumption. A soda every once in a while, sure that's understandable; however, having one or two sodas every single day is something that can be detrimental to your health in the long-run.

Gluten-Free Eating

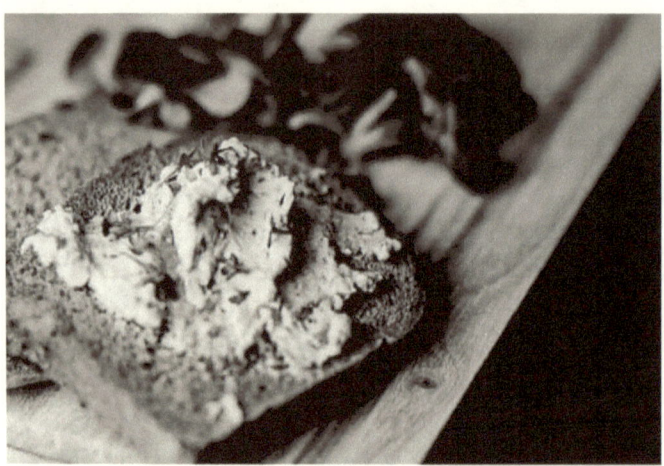

The next topic is one that is currently somewhat of a trend. Yes, this is the topic of the gluten-free diet. The gluten-free diet seemed to become more popular after the release of the book *Wheat Belly*, which was all about how wheat as a plant has changed in composition over the years and is no longer the same type of wheat that our ancestors digested.

For these reasons and many others, it's best to stay away from it. Now, I'm not too sure about the legitimacy of the claims that were made in the book *Wheat Belly*; however, I can attest to the fact that going completely gluten-free does lead to a flatter stomach. What's more, you are still able to eat many types of delicious

foods if you are sticking to a gluten-free diet but you're not worried about keeping other types of dieting goals in check. For example, if you decide to become gluten-free but not necessarily health-conscious, this might mean that you choose to indulge in French fries every once in a while.

It also means that you can treat yourself to ice cream, too. If you decide to go gluten-free, make sure that you're not purchasing those gluten-free products that you can find at specialty markets such as Whole Foods or Rastelli's. While these products are convenient, they're also often laced with the same number of carbs and sugar that can be found in gluten-laden products.

Moderation

For all of the healthy eating habits that we've discussed in this chapter, a common thread that runs through all of them is the idea that you need to be partaking in these dietary restrictions in moderation.

Of course, if you decide that you're going to be a vegetarian or a vegan, there is not much moderation within this. You are either all in, or you're not. For the other types of healthy eating that we've discussed, however, it's important that you pat yourself on the back every so often and admire any progress that you've made. No one likes to hear their friends whine and complain about their terrible diet. Make exceptions for yourself. Eat the cake every once in a while. As long as you work hard

during your workouts and push your body to new limits,
it's going to be okay.

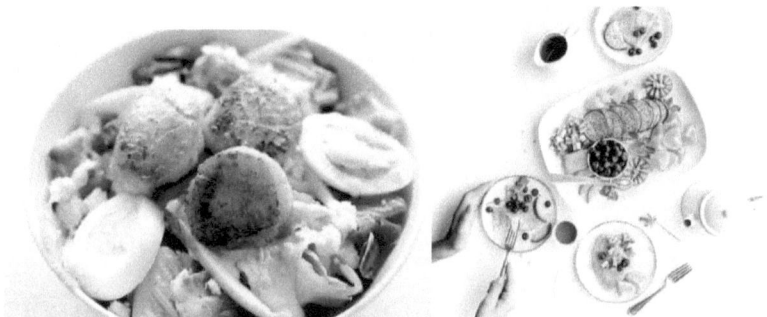

Chapter 10: Success Story about the At~Home At~Work Workout Method

You have most of the information that you need in order to successfully transition to a healthier and more active lifestyle for yourself, all except for one piece of the puzzle. This piece is known as motivation.

Let's take a look at a success story that will help you to see that results through the home and work exercise regime is entirely possible. After you've heard about the success of others, you'll be able to go out there and find some success for yourself

Meet Jenn !

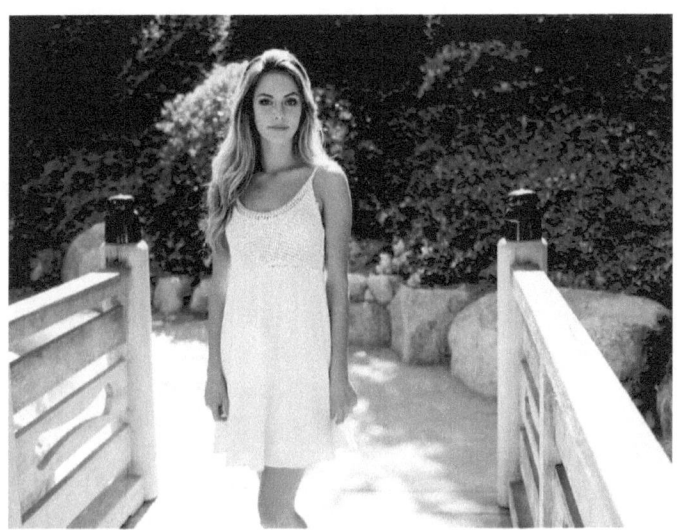

Jenn was already a pretty fit woman, but after going through her first pregnancy, she came back to work realizing that her body had become rather unattractive and frumpy. Of course, to her husband her body looked perfectly fine.

Jenn felt frumpy and unhappy because of her own body standards.

You see, Jenn grew up participating in gymnastics and even acrobats for a short time. She had been fit for most of her life, so the weight gain certainly did not make Jenn feel happy or confident about herself. Not wanting to continue on this path, Jenn decided that she was going to do something to change the path of her future weight.

With diapers and childcare being so expensive, Jenn knew that she would likely not have time to go to a gym three times a week. Both her and her husband had full time jobs. With a new baby in the house, she didn't see a way to make this possible. Instead, Jenn decided that she was going to learn about how she could start exercising at work. She also supplemented this with yoga and Pilates at home when she wasn't being consumed with mommy duties.

She dedicated herself to clean eating, and got down to it. Within three months Jenn had lost most of the baby weight that she had gained during her pregnancy. While this was certainly impressive, what was even more impressive was the fact that she had inspired others around her in her office to also desire better fitness for themselves. She ended up eventually organizing an office walk-a-thon at her place of work for her and her employees.

She even convinced her company to allow a yoga instructor to come to the office once a month on the company dime. While yoga once a month is not that much yoga, it still gave people who typically did not participate with yoga exposure to the practice. Jenn did all of this without much money. What she had mostly was a desire to better herself and her physical circumstances.

This proved to be enough to better the lives of her fellow employees and her overall office culture as well. Who knows what you'll be able to do if you can find it within yourself to start exercising in the ways that have been presented in this book. Maybe you'll even be able to extend your workout goals to others around you. If you don't try, you'll have no way of knowing how far you can go.

Hopefully Jenn's story has provided you with the motivation that you need to jump into your own at-home or at-work work out head first! All of the other information that you need has been presented in the previous chapters of this book. Taking action based on this information, now that's on you to achieve for yourself.

Conclusion

Thank for making it through to the end of *At-Home At-Work Workouts 365: The Most Effective, Convenient and FREE Workouts on the Planet and Get Ultimate Results*, let's hope it was informative and able to provide you with all of the tools you need to achieve your goals whatever it may be.

The next step is to start trying these workouts for yourself! If you're someone who would like to keep their workouts more private than public, this means that you should first start trying out these workouts and breathing exercises at home rather than in the workplace. After you get used to the workouts and feel confident about how they're making you feel, you can then expand your workout regime to include the workplace.

If you don't care about how you're perceived by others in the workplace, then you should start trying these workouts in both places! Who knows, maybe someone at your office will end up wanting to workout with you. If you find someone who is eager and willing to do this, you two can better yourselves together. It's always nice to have a partner who is by your side, pushing you to improve yourself as they expect you to push them too.

Finally, if you found this book useful in anyway, a review on Amazon is always appreciated!